HIGH TRIGLYCERIDES DIET HANDBOOK

1500 Days' Worth Of Heart-Healthy, Triglyceride-Lowering Recipes (38-Day Meal Plan)

Vanessa Meza

Table of Contents

INTRODUCTION TO HIGH TRIGLYCERIDES DIET

A. Explanation Of High Triglycerides

B. Importance Of Diet In Managing Triglyceride Levels

C. Purpose And Scope Of The Book

A. Explanation of High Triglycerides:

Definition: Triglycerides are a type of fat (lipid) found in your blood. When you eat, your body converts any calories it doesn't need to use right away into triglycerides. These triglycerides are stored in your fat cells for later use. However, consistently high levels of triglycerides in your blood can increase your risk of heart disease, stroke, and other health problems.

Causes: High triglyceride levels can be caused by various factors, including genetics, lifestyle choices (such as diet and physical activity levels), certain medical conditions (such as diabetes, obesity, and thyroid disorders), and medications (such as steroids, birth control pills, and diuretics).

Symptoms: High triglycerides typically don't cause any symptoms on their own. They are usually detected through blood tests ordered by a healthcare provider. However, extremely high levels can sometimes cause symptoms such as pancreatitis (inflammation of the pancreas), abdominal pain, and fatty deposits on the skin.

Health Risks: Elevated triglyceride levels are often associated with other risk factors for heart disease, such as high LDL cholesterol, low HDL cholesterol, high blood pressure, and insulin resistance. Managing triglyceride levels is important for overall heart health.

B. Importance of Diet in Managing Triglyceride Levels:

Role of Diet: Diet plays a crucial role in managing triglyceride levels. Certain dietary choices can either raise or lower triglyceride levels in the blood.

Foods to Limit: Foods high in sugars and refined carbohydrates can significantly increase triglyceride levels. This includes sugary beverages, sweets, white bread, pasta, and other processed foods. Also, consuming excessive amounts of alcohol can raise triglyceride levels.

Foods to Include: A heart-healthy diet that includes plenty of fruits, vegetables, whole grains, lean proteins (such as fish, poultry, and legumes), and healthy fats (such as those found in nuts, seeds, and olive oil) can help lower triglyceride levels. Omega-3 fatty acids, found in fatty fish like salmon and mackerel, have been shown to reduce triglycerides.

Portion Control and Balanced Eating: Managing portion sizes and eating balanced meals throughout the day can also help stabilize triglyceride levels. Avoiding large meals and excessive snacking can prevent spikes in triglycerides after eating.

Lifestyle Changes: In addition to dietary changes, maintaining a healthy weight, engaging in regular physical activity, quitting smoking, and managing stress are important lifestyle factors for managing triglyceride levels.

C. Purpose and Scope of the Book:

Purpose: The purpose of the book is to provide comprehensive information and practical guidance on understanding, managing, and lowering high triglyceride levels to improve heart health and overall well-being.

Scope: The book covers various aspects related to high triglycerides, including their causes, health risks, diagnosis, treatment options, lifestyle modifications, and dietary strategies. It aims to empower readers with the knowledge and tools they need to take control of their triglyceride levels and reduce their risk of cardiovascular disease.

Audience: The book is intended for a general audience interested in learning more about heart health and managing triglyceride levels. It may be particularly useful for individuals with elevated triglycerides or those at risk of developing heart disease, as well as healthcare professionals looking to deepen their understanding of this topic.

CHAPTER ONE

UNDERSTANDING TRIGLYCERIDES

A. What Are Triglycerides?

B. Causes And Risk Factors

C. Health Implications Of High Triglycerides

A. What are Triglycerides?

Definition: Triglycerides are a type of fat (lipid) found in your blood. They are the most common type of fat in the body and serve as a major source of energy. When you eat, your body converts any calories it doesn't need to use immediately into triglycerides. These triglycerides are then stored in fat cells throughout the body.

Chemical Structure: Triglycerides consist of three fatty acid molecules attached to a glycerol molecule. This structure allows them to be easily transported through the bloodstream to cells where they can be used for energy.

Functions: Triglycerides play several important roles in the body, including providing energy for cellular function, insulating and protecting organs, and serving as a source of essential fatty acids that are necessary for various bodily processes.

B. Causes and Risk Factors:

Dietary Factors: Consumption of foods high in sugars, refined carbohydrates, and unhealthy fats can increase triglyceride levels in the blood. This includes foods like sugary beverages, sweets, fried foods, processed snacks, and high-fat dairy products.

Lifestyle Choices: Sedentary lifestyle, lack of physical activity, and excess weight or obesity can contribute to elevated triglyceride levels. Regular physical activity helps to lower triglycerides by burning excess fat and improving insulin sensitivity.

Genetic Factors: Some individuals may have a genetic predisposition to high triglyceride levels. Certain genetic disorders, such as familial hypertriglyceridemia, can lead to extremely high triglyceride levels even in the absence of other risk factors.

Medical Conditions: Certain medical conditions and health issues can also increase triglyceride levels. These include type 2 diabetes, metabolic syndrome, hypothyroidism, kidney disease, and liver disease.

Medications: Some medications can raise triglyceride levels as a side effect.

These may include certain types of diuretics, beta-blockers, corticosteroids, estrogen-containing drugs (such as birth control pills), and immunosuppressants.

C. Health Implications of High Triglycerides:

Cardiovascular Disease: Elevated triglyceride levels are associated with an increased risk of cardiovascular disease, including heart attack, stroke, and atherosclerosis (hardening and narrowing of the arteries).

Pancreatitis: Extremely high levels of triglycerides can lead to acute pancreatitis, a painful inflammation of the pancreas. This condition requires immediate medical attention and can be life-threatening if not treated promptly.

Metabolic Syndrome: High triglyceride levels are often a component of metabolic syndrome, a cluster of conditions that increase the risk of heart disease, stroke, and type 2 diabetes. Other components of metabolic syndrome include abdominal obesity, high blood pressure, and insulin resistance.

Non-Alcoholic Fatty Liver Disease (NAFLD): Elevated triglyceride levels are associated with an increased risk of NAFLD, a condition characterized by excessive fat accumulation in the liver. NAFLD can progress to more severe liver damage, including non-alcoholic steatohepatitis (NASH) and cirrhosis.

CHAPTER TWO

THE ROLE OF DIET IN MANAGING TRIGLYCERIDES

A. Impact Of Dietary Choices On Triglyceride Levels

B. Key Nutritional Components For Triglyceride Management

C. Foods To Avoid And Foods To Include

A. Impact of Dietary Choices on Triglyceride Levels:

Sugars and Refined Carbohydrates: Foods high in sugars and refined carbohydrates can cause a rapid increase in triglyceride levels. This includes sugary beverages, sweets, pastries, white bread, pasta, and other processed foods made with white flour.

Unhealthy Fats: Trans fats and saturated fats found in fried foods, processed snacks, red meat, and full-fat dairy products can also elevate triglyceride levels.

Alcohol: Excessive alcohol consumption can significantly raise triglyceride levels, especially in individuals predisposed to hypertriglyceridemia. Alcohol is metabolized in the liver, leading to increased triglyceride production and decreased triglyceride clearance from the bloodstream.

B. Key Nutritional Components for Triglyceride Management:

Omega-3 Fatty Acids: Omega-3 fatty acids, found primarily in fatty fish such as salmon, mackerel, sardines, and trout, are known to lower triglyceride levels. They can also be obtained from plant-based sources like flaxseeds, chia seeds, walnuts, and hemp seeds.

Monounsaturated Fats: Foods rich in monounsaturated fats, such as olive oil, avocados, and nuts (like almonds, peanuts, and cashews), can help lower triglycerides and improve heart health.

Fiber: Soluble fiber found in fruits, vegetables, whole grains, legumes, and oats can help reduce triglyceride levels by slowing down the absorption of sugars and fats in the digestive tract.

Lean Proteins: Lean protein sources, such as poultry, fish, tofu, and legumes, are important components of a triglyceride-lowering diet. They provide essential nutrients without adding excess saturated fats or cholesterol.

C. Foods to Avoid and Foods to Include:

Foods to Avoid:

Sugary beverages: Regular consumption of sugary drinks like soda and fruit juices can significantly raise triglyceride levels.

Sweets and desserts: Limit intake of candies, cookies, cakes, and other high-sugar treats.

Fried foods: Avoid fried foods like french fries, fried chicken, and doughnuts, which are high in unhealthy fats.

Processed snacks: Snack foods like chips, crackers, and cookies often contain unhealthy fats and refined carbohydrates.

High-fat dairy products: Opt for low-fat or fat-free dairy options to reduce saturated fat intake.

Excessive alcohol: Limit alcohol consumption to moderate levels (if at all) to help maintain healthy triglyceride levels.

Foods to Include:

Fatty fish: Incorporate fatty fish into your diet at least twice a week to benefit from omega-3 fatty acids.

Fruits and vegetables: Aim to fill half your plate with colorful fruits and vegetables, which is rich in fiber and antioxidants.

Whole grains: Choose whole grains like brown rice, quinoa, barley, and whole wheat bread over refined grains.

Nuts and seeds: Enjoy a handful of nuts or seeds as a snack or add them to salads, yogurt, or oatmeal for a heart-healthy boost.

Olive oil: Use olive oil as your primary cooking oil or drizzle it over salads and vegetables for added flavor and monounsaturated fats.

Legumes: Incorporate beans, lentils, and chickpeas into soups, stews, salads, and side dishes for plant-based protein and fiber.

DESIGNING YOUR HIGH TRIGLYCERIDES DIET PLAN

A. Assessing Current Dietary Habits:

Food Diary: Start by keeping a detailed food diary for a few days to track everything you eat and drink. This will provide insight into your current dietary habits, including patterns of food consumption, portion sizes, and food choices.

Identify Triglyceride Triggers: Review your food diary to identify specific dietary factors that may be contributing to elevated triglyceride levels, such as consumption of sugary foods and drinks, refined carbohydrates, unhealthy fats, and excessive alcohol.

Assess Nutrient Intake: Evaluate your intake of key nutrients known to influence triglyceride levels, including omega-3 fatty acids, monounsaturated fats, fiber, and lean proteins. Determine whether your diet is balanced and provides adequate amounts of these nutrients.

B. Setting Realistic Goals:

Consult Healthcare Provider: Discuss your triglyceride levels and dietary goals with your healthcare provider or a registered dietitian. They can provide personalized guidance and help you set realistic and achievable goals based on your individual health status, preferences, and lifestyle.

SMART Goals: Set Specific, Measurable, Achievable, Relevant, and Time-bound (SMART) goals for improving your diet and managing triglyceride levels. For example, aim to reduce consumption of sugary beverages to no more than one per day within the next month.

Gradual Changes: Start with small, achievable changes to your diet rather than trying to overhaul your eating habits all at once. Gradual changes are more sustainable and easier to maintain over the long term.

C. Creating a Balanced and Sustainable Diet Plan:

Focus on Whole Foods: Base your diet around whole, minimally processed foods, including fruits, vegetables, whole grains, lean proteins, and healthy fats. These foods provide essential nutrients and are generally lower in unhealthy fats, sugars, and refined carbohydrates.

Portion Control: Pay attention to portion sizes and avoid oversized servings, especially of calorie-dense foods. Use smaller plates, bowls, and utensils to help control portion sizes and prevent overeating.

Meal Planning: Plan your meals and snacks in advance to ensure you have nutritious options readily available.

Include a variety of foods from all food groups to ensure a balanced intake of nutrients.

Include Triglyceride-Lowering Foods: Incorporate foods known to help lower triglyceride levels, such as fatty fish (rich in omega-3 fatty acids), fruits, vegetables, whole grains, nuts, seeds, and legumes.

Limit Triglyceride-Raising Foods: Reduce intake of foods that can elevate triglyceride levels, including sugary beverages, sweets, refined carbohydrates, fried foods, processed snacks, high-fat dairy products, and excessive alcohol.

Hydration: Stay hydrated by drinking plenty of water throughout the day. Water is essential for overall health and can help support optimal metabolism and nutrient absorption.

IMPLEMENTING YOUR DIET PLAN

A. Practical Tips For Grocery Shopping

B. Meal Planning Strategies

C. Incorporating Exercise For Enhanced Results

A. Practical Tips for Grocery Shopping:

Make a List: Before heading to the grocery store, make a list of the foods you need based on your meal plan and dietary goals. Stick to your list to avoid impulse purchases of unhealthy items.

Shop the Perimeter: Focus on shopping around the perimeter of the grocery store, where fresh produce, lean proteins, dairy, and whole grains are typically located. Limit time spent in the aisles containing processed and packaged foods.

Read Labels: Take time to read nutrition labels and ingredient lists on packaged foods. Look for products with lower amounts of added sugars, unhealthy fats (saturated and trans fats), and sodium.

Choose Fresh and Whole Foods: Opt for fresh fruits and vegetables, whole grains (such as brown rice, quinoa, and oats), lean meats (like poultry and fish), low-fat dairy products, and unsalted nuts and seeds.

Stock Up on Healthy Staples: Keep your kitchen stocked with pantry staples like beans, lentils, canned tomatoes, whole-grain pasta, and healthy cooking oils (like olive oil) to make nutritious meals at home.

B. **Meal Planning Strategies**:

Plan Ahead: Set aside time each week to plan your meals and snacks for the upcoming days. Consider your schedule, dietary preferences, and any special occasions or events.

Batch Cooking: Cook large batches of staple foods like grains, beans, and proteins on your meal prep day to use throughout the week. This can save time and make it easier to assemble meals on busy days.

Prep Ingredients: Wash, chop, and portion out fruits, vegetables, and other ingredients in advance to streamline meal preparation. Store prepped ingredients in airtight containers in the refrigerator for easy access.

Mix and Match: Create a flexible meal plan that allows you to mix and match ingredients to make a variety of meals. For example, cook a batch of grilled chicken breast and use it in salads, stir-fries, wraps, and pasta dishes throughout the week.

Include Quick and Easy Options: Plan for simple meals and snacks that require minimal preparation, such as smoothies, salads, sandwiches, and yogurt with fruit and nuts.

C. Incorporating Exercise for Enhanced Results:

Aerobic Exercise: Engage in regular aerobic exercise, such as walking, jogging, cycling, swimming, or dancing, to help lower triglyceride levels and improve cardiovascular health. Aim for at least 150 minutes of moderate-intensity aerobic activity per week.

Strength Training: Incorporate strength training exercises into your routine to build muscle mass and boost metabolism. Include exercises that target major muscle groups, such as squats, lunges, push-ups, and rows, at least two days per week.

Interval Training: Consider incorporating interval training, which alternates between high-intensity bursts of activity and periods of rest or lower intensity. This can be an effective way to burn calories, improve fitness, and lower triglyceride levels.

Stay Active Throughout the Day: Look for opportunities to increase your daily activity level by taking the stairs instead of the elevator, parking farther away from your destination, or taking short activity breaks throughout the day.

Find Activities You Enjoy: Choose activities and exercises that you enjoy and that fit your lifestyle and preferences. Whether it's dancing, hiking, gardening, or playing a sport, finding activities you love can make exercise more enjoyable and sustainable.

RECIPES AND MEAL IDEAS

A. Breakfast Options

B. Lunch Suggestions C. Dinner Recipes

D. Snack Ideas

A. Breakfast Options:

Greek Yogurt Parfait: Layer Greek yogurt with fresh berries, sliced bananas, and a sprinkle of granola or chopped nuts for added crunch and flavor.

Vegetable Omelette: Whisk together eggs with diced bell peppers, onions, spinach, and a sprinkle of cheese. Cook in a skillet until set and serve with whole-grain toast.

Overnight Oats: Combine rolled oats with milk (or yogurt), chia seeds, and your choice of flavorings such as vanilla extract, cinnamon, and honey. Let it sit in the refrigerator overnight and top with sliced fruit in the morning.

Avocado Toast: Mash ripe avocado onto whole-grain toast and top with sliced tomatoes, a drizzle of olive oil, and a sprinkle of salt and pepper.

Smoothie Bowl: Blend together frozen mixed berries, banana, spinach, and Greek yogurt until smooth. Pour into a bowl and top with sliced fruit, nuts, seeds, and a drizzle of honey.

B. Lunch Suggestions:

Quinoa Salad: Toss cooked quinoa with chopped vegetables (such as cucumber, bell peppers, cherry tomatoes, and red onion) and fresh herbs. Dress with a simple vinaigrette made with olive oil, lemon juice, and Dijon mustard.

Grilled Chicken Wrap: Fill a whole-grain wrap with grilled chicken breast, mixed greens, sliced avocado, and hummus. Roll it up and serve with carrot sticks and cucumber slices.

Mediterranean Chickpea Salad: Combine cooked chickpeas with diced cucumber, cherry tomatoes, red onion, feta cheese, Kalamata olives, and chopped parsley. Dress with olive oil, lemon juice, garlic, and oregano.

Vegetable Stir-Fry: Stir-fry a mix of colorful vegetables (such as broccoli, bell peppers, snap peas, carrots, and mushrooms) in a light sauce made with soy sauce, ginger, and garlic. Serve over brown rice or quinoa.

Turkey and Veggie Wrap: Fill a whole-grain wrap with sliced turkey breast, lettuce, tomato, cucumber, and a smear of hummus or avocado. Serve with a side of baby carrots and hummus.

C. Dinner Recipes:

Baked Salmon: Season salmon fillets with olive oil, lemon juice, garlic, and herbs. Bake in the oven until cooked through and serve with steamed broccoli and quinoa pilaf.

Vegetable and Lentil Curry: Simmer lentils with diced vegetables (such as cauliflower, bell peppers, and spinach) in a flavorful curry sauce made with coconut milk, ginger, garlic, and curry spices. Serve over brown rice.

Grilled Vegetable Skewers: Thread skewers with a variety of colorful vegetables (such as cherry tomatoes, zucchini, mushrooms, bell peppers, and red onion) marinated in olive oil, balsamic vinegar, and herbs. Grill until tender and serve with couscous.

Turkey Chili: Cook ground turkey with diced onions, bell peppers, garlic, and chili spices in a pot. Add canned tomatoes, kidney beans, and corn, and simmer until flavors meld. Serve with a dollop of Greek yogurt and a sprinkle of cheese.

Stuffed Bell Peppers: Fill halved bell peppers with a mixture of cooked quinoa, black beans, corn, diced tomatoes, and spices. Top with cheese and bake until peppers are tender.

D. Snack Ideas:

Apple Slices with Almond Butter: Spread almond butter onto apple slices for a satisfying and nutritious snack.

Greek Yogurt with Berries: Enjoy a serving of Greek yogurt topped with fresh berries for a protein-rich snack.

Hummus and Veggie Sticks: Dip carrot, celery, cucumber, and bell pepper sticks into hummus for a crunchy and flavorful snack.

Trail Mix: Mix together nuts, seeds, dried fruit, and a sprinkle of dark chocolate chips for a portable and energizing snack.

Whole Grain Crackers with Avocado: Top whole-grain crackers with mashed avocado and a sprinkle of sea salt for a quick and healthy snack.

OVERCOMING CHALLENGES AND STAYING MOTIVATED

A. Dealing With Cravings

B. Handling Social Situations

C. Tracking Progress And Adjusting Your Plan

A. Dealing with Cravings:

Identify Triggers: Pay attention to what triggers your cravings, whether it's stress, boredom, emotions, or specific food cues. Understanding your triggers can help you develop strategies to manage cravings more effectively.

Plan Ahead: Anticipate situations where cravings are likely to occur, such as during times of stress or when you're surrounded by tempting foods. Plan ahead by having healthier alternatives available to satisfy cravings.

Choose Healthier Options: When cravings strike, opt for healthier alternatives that still satisfy your taste buds. For example, if you're craving something sweet, reach for a piece of fruit or a small serving of dark chocolate.

Practice Mindful Eating: Slow down and pay attention to your eating experience, focusing on the flavors, textures, and sensations of each bite. Mindful eating can help you become more aware of your body's hunger and fullness cues, making it easier to manage cravings.

Stay Hydrated: Drink plenty of water throughout the day, as dehydration can sometimes be mistaken for hunger. Keep a water bottle handy and take sips regularly to stay hydrated and curb cravings.

B. Handling Social Situations:

Communicate Your Goals: Be open with friends and family about your dietary goals and the importance of managing your triglyceride levels. Explain your reasons for making healthier choices and ask for their support.

Offer to Bring a Dish: If you're attending a social gathering or potluck, offer to bring a nutritious dish that aligns with your dietary goals. This ensures that you'll have a healthier option available to enjoy.

Focus on Socializing: Shift the focus away from food by engaging in activities that don't revolve around eating, such as going for a walk, playing games, or having meaningful conversations.

Practice Assertiveness: Don't feel pressured to eat foods that don't align with your dietary goals. Politely decline offerings or suggest alternative options that you feel comfortable with.

Be Flexible: While it's important to stick to your dietary plan as much as possible, it's also okay to indulge occasionally in moderation. Allow yourself to enjoy special occasions and social gatherings without feeling guilty.

C. Tracking Progress and Adjusting Your Plan:

Keep a Food Diary: Track your food intake, including meals, snacks, and beverages, to monitor your progress and identify areas for improvement. This can help you stay accountable and make adjustments as needed.

Monitor Triglyceride Levels: Work with your healthcare provider to regularly monitor your triglyceride levels through blood tests. Use these results to gauge the effectiveness of your diet plan and make necessary adjustments.

Set Milestones: Break down your goals into smaller, achievable milestones and celebrate your progress along the way. This can help keep you motivated and focused on your long-term success.

Be Flexible: Recognize that your dietary needs and preferences may change over time, and be willing to adapt your plan accordingly. Stay open to trying new foods, recipes, and strategies to find what works best for you.

Seek Support: Don't hesitate to reach out for support from friends, family, or a healthcare professional if you're struggling to stay motivated or make progress. Having a support system can provide encouragement and accountability.

CHAPTER THREE

BEYOND DIET: LIFESTYLE FACTORS FOR TRIGLYCERIDE MANAGEMENT

A. Importance Of Stress Management

B. Getting Sufficient Sleep

C. Limiting Alcohol Consumption

A. Importance of Stress Management:

Effect on Triglycerides: Chronic stress can lead to elevated triglyceride levels by triggering the release of stress hormones like cortisol, which can increase the production of triglycerides in the liver.

Impact on Lifestyle Choices: Stress can also influence dietary habits and lifestyle choices, leading to increased consumption of unhealthy foods, emotional eating, and decreased physical activity, all of which can contribute to higher triglyceride levels.

Stress Reduction Techniques: Incorporate stress reduction techniques into your daily routine, such as mindfulness meditation, deep breathing exercises, yoga, tai chi, or spending time in nature. These practices can help lower stress levels and improve overall well-being.

B. Getting Sufficient Sleep:

Role in Metabolism: Adequate sleep is essential for regulating metabolism and maintaining hormonal balance, including hormones that influence appetite, food intake, and lipid metabolism.

Effects on Triglycerides: Lack of sleep or poor sleep quality can disrupt metabolic processes and lead to dysregulation of lipid metabolism, potentially increasing triglyceride levels.

Recommendations: Aim for 7-9 hours of quality sleep per night to support overall health and help manage triglyceride levels. Establish a consistent sleep schedule, create a relaxing bedtime routine, and optimize your sleep environment for restful sleep.

C. Limiting Alcohol Consumption: Impact on Triglycerides: Excessive alcohol consumption can significantly raise triglyceride levels by increasing the production of triglycerides in the liver and impairing their clearance from the bloodstream.

Moderate Alcohol Intake: If you choose to drink alcohol, do so in moderation. For most adults, moderate alcohol consumption is defined as up to one drink per day for women and up to two drinks per day for men.

Healthy Alternatives: Opt for healthier alternatives to alcohol, such as sparkling water with a splash of citrus juice or herbal tea, to reduce overall alcohol intake and minimize its impact on triglyceride levels.

Be Mindful of Mixers: Be mindful of high-sugar mixers and cocktails, as they can contribute to increased triglyceride levels. Choose low-sugar or sugar-free mixers and limit added sugars in drinks.

CHAPTER FOUR

SEEKING PROFESSIONAL GUIDANCE

A. When to Consult a Healthcare Provider:

High Triglyceride Levels: If you have high triglyceride levels or a family history of high triglycerides and related health issues, such as cardiovascular disease, it's important to consult a healthcare provider for evaluation and management.

Risk Factors: If you have risk factors for high triglycerides, such as obesity, diabetes, metabolic syndrome, or a sedentary lifestyle, consider discussing your concerns with a healthcare provider to assess your risk and develop a plan for prevention or treatment.

Symptoms: If you experience symptoms related to high triglycerides, such as abdominal pain, pancreatitis, or fatty deposits on the skin, seek prompt medical attention from a healthcare provider.

B. Working with a Registered Dietitian:

Personalized Nutrition Guidance: A registered dietitian (RD) can provide personalized nutrition guidance tailored to your individual needs, preferences, and health goals.

Dietary Assessment: An RD can conduct a thorough dietary assessment to evaluate your current eating habits, identify areas for improvement, and develop a customized diet plan to help manage high triglycerides.

Education and Support: RDs can educate you about the role of diet in managing triglyceride levels, teach you how to make healthier food choices, and provide ongoing support and accountability as you work towards your goals.

Nutrition Counseling: Nutrition counseling sessions with an RD can help you overcome challenges, address barriers to success, and make sustainable lifestyle changes to improve your overall health and well-being.

C. Utilizing Support Groups and Resources:

Support Groups: Consider joining support groups or online communities focused on heart health, nutrition, and managing high triglycerides. These groups can provide valuable support, encouragement, and shared experiences with others facing similar challenges.

Educational Resources: Take advantage of educational resources provided by reputable organizations, such as the American Heart Association, National Lipid Association, and Academy of Nutrition and Dietetics. These resources may include articles, fact sheets, recipes, and online tools to help you learn more about managing high triglycerides.

Community Programs: Look for community programs or workshops that offer education and support for individuals with high triglycerides or other cardiovascular risk factors. These programs may include group classes, cooking demonstrations, and lifestyle coaching to help you implement healthy changes.

CONCLUSION

A. Recap of Key Points:

High triglyceride levels are a common lipid disorder that can increase the risk of cardiovascular disease and other health complications.

Dietary choices play a significant role in managing triglyceride levels, with a focus on consuming whole foods, healthy fats, lean proteins, fiber-rich foods, and limiting sugars, refined carbohydrates, and unhealthy fats.

Lifestyle factors such as stress management, sufficient sleep, and moderate alcohol consumption also influence triglyceride levels and overall heart health.

Seeking professional guidance from healthcare providers and registered dietitians, and utilizing support groups and educational resources, can provide valuable support and guidance in managing high triglycerides.

B. Encouragement for Long-Term Success:

Managing high triglycerides requires commitment, patience, and consistency. Small, sustainable changes made over time can lead to significant improvements in triglyceride levels and overall health.

Celebrate your successes, no matter how small, and recognize the progress you've made towards your health goals. Each positive choice you make brings you closer to long-term success.

Remember that setbacks are a natural part of the journey. If you experience challenges or setbacks along the way, don't be discouraged. Use them as opportunities to learn, grow, and recommit to your health goals.

C. Empowerment to Take Control of Your Health Journey:

You have the power to take control of your health journey and make positive changes to manage high triglycerides and improve your overall well-being.

Educate yourself about the role of diet, lifestyle factors, and other interventions in managing triglyceride levels. Knowledge is empowering and can help you make informed decisions about your health.

Advocate for yourself and actively participate in your healthcare by seeking professional guidance, asking questions, and collaborating with healthcare providers and registered dietitians to develop a personalized plan that meets your needs and goals.

Remember that you are capable, resilient, and deserving of good health. By prioritizing self-care, making positive choices, and staying committed to your health journey, you can achieve long-term success in managing high triglycerides and living your best life.

THE END